Introduction To The Author

Hello. My name is Jamie Valencia Wilkinson (Wilkinson-Watson). I am a student at Harvard University and a stay-at-home married, mother of two beautiful children.

Throughout my life I have tried many things-- vegetarianism being one of them. Natural foods and their composition have increased the quality of my health tremendously.

Throughout my book, I hope to discuss these beneficial effects in a concise and conversational manner. Have fun!

Types of Medicine

In The Bahamas, there are many traditions that are upheld each and every year. One of these is the use of alternative medicine.

While many people around the world have no idea what the heck herbal medicines are, many people still do.

Let us first take a look at the types of remedies.

There are two kinds of medicine:

Man-made- these are synthetic pharmaceuticals that are as the name suggests artificial. They are usually created within a laboratory setting.

Herbal Medicine (and fruits and vegetables)- these are medicines that are derived from nature. They usually have little to no side effects.

*Medicines are the things we take to feel better or be healthy.

Herbs (and fruits and vegetables) belong to the plant kingdom and they have two types of names—a scientific and a common name.

For instance, the common Aloe(s) plant is known by its scientific name Aloe vera. The first part of its nomenclature has an uppercase letter and the second part of it has a lowercase letter. Also, it is normally or sometimes italicized when printed in encyclopedias, journals, etc.

Throughout this text, we will be using both names interchangeablely. Feel free to look up the scienitific names of each plant for your own edification.

<u>Reiteration-What are medicines?</u>

So let us reiterate the fact that medicines are those things that we take in order to feel better whenever, we are ill (or trying to prevent sickness). Sometimes, it is important to consider the fact that there are no known cures for every disease out there.

Therefore, we must remember to use the terms treat and cure accordingly—because they are totally different.

Here is a small list of herbal medicine:

Aloe vera

Sun Flower

Licorice

Dill

Eucalyptus

Cinnamon

Fever Grass

Catnip

Ginseng

Shepherd's Needle

<u>Aloe vera</u>

Aloe is a green, luscious plant with a very bitter taste. It is extremely good for your skin and body.

It:

-reduces cancer

- minimizes constipation and other digestive problems

- it treats the flu and the common cold

- and it treats wounds, cuts and acne

<u>Sunflower</u>

Sunflowers are just so beautiful aren't they? They have golden petals and their seeds are rich in nutrition.

This plant has the ability to filter out harmful, cancer inducing, radioactive waste from your soil and aquifers.

Plant a few of these in your backyard because doing so can also improve your air quality.

Licorice

When you pronounce the word "licorice", you automatically think about candy. However, it is not candy. Instead, it is a powerful plant that can:

- boost your immune system
- treat respiratory ailments like asthma
- help with digestive disturbances (it is a laxative)
- etc.

There have been speculation that it can slow down the effects of HIV and herpes (Livestrong.com).

Dill

Dill and its seed is most commonly used on infants and babies. However, adults can use it too because of its anti-bacterial and anti-carcinogenic properties.

Eucalyptus

Eucalyptus is excellent for your skin. It is an ingredient in some of the top selling skin cleansers.

<u>Cinnamon</u>

Not only is it good for seasoning desserts and other foods but cinnamon can also be used to treat the flu and cold.

Fever Grass

Fever grass is as its name suggests, used to treat or stabilize a fever. Fevers occur when the body is trying to fight off an infection. The normal body temperature is 98.6 degrees fahrenheit.

<u>Catnip</u>

The felines go crazy for it! Catnip is a very versatile herb. It can be used for:

- mosquito repellant

- sleep

- sedative

-etc

Ginseng

Ginseng has been known to:

- boost the sex drive

- keep an individual energized

- promote good brain function

- lower blood sugar (newsmax.com)

- etc.

Shepherd's Needle

It is said to treat stomach ailments and fevers.

The Nutritional Value of Fruits and Vegetables/The Benefits of Vegetaranism

In the past I have managed to stay on the vegan/vegetarian diet for five years. During that time, I had no meat to eat-- not even eggs.

Throughout the weeks and months, my body changed dramatically. I started to lose weight, my immune system was better, my hair grew more (because of less sugar), my bowel movements became regular and my skin glowed. My body was literally cleaning itself out.

My acne began to disappear and I felt very energetic all the time. I felt good on the inside and outside.

The only bad part about all of that is that your body needs vitamin B12, and research shows that it is only present in meat.Some other studies claim that it can be found in seaweed.

And lets be real-- you will get the ocassional meat craving from time to time.

<u>Apple</u>

Apples are rich in fiber and vitamin C. Apples also fight cancer forming cells.

<u>Orange</u>

Oranges are tangy, juicy and full of vitamins C and E. It is known to make your skin glow.

<u>Grape</u>

Grapes are an excellent source of phytochemicals. They are very delicious and nutritious. They have a very beautiful colour and destroy oxygen free radicals.

<u>Blueberry</u>

This fruit is very dark in color-- and has alot of flavonoids. It is good for cleansing the kidneys, fighting off infection and the cold and flu.

<u>Horseradish</u>

Horseradishes are antibacterial in nature and they are a very significant source of vitamin C.

<u>Celery</u>

Alot of people don't know that celery is excellent in fighting off cancer cells. It is green which means that it is rich in vitamin D.

<u>Tomatoes</u>

Tomatoes are rich in vitamin C, lycopene, and vitamin E. These vitamins promote good skin health and also fight off disease.

Onion

Like garlic, onion also has a rather offensive smell. Additionally, it is said to fight off the flu and common cold.

Garlic

Garlic, with its pungent smell, is one of the most effective herbs out there for fighting disease.

It has anti- viral properties, it fights of bacteria and it is even said to destroy cancer-causing cells.

Preventative Tips To Avoid Disease, Ailments And Infections

- Always wash your hands

- Breathe fresh air

- Wash foods such as fruits, vegetables and meat

- Brush your teeth and floss

- Drink a lot of water

- Be active; exercise or walk as much as possible

- Think good thoughts

- Find inner peace and comfort

- Set goals for yourself and accomplish them

- Smile

- Use honey as a substitute instead of using sugar

- Take your vitamins

- Get some sunlight

- Enjoy a fruit and vegetable smoothie sometimes

- Maintain an excellent circadian/sleeping cycle

- Have a proper diet

- Use the bathroom on time

Conclusion

Foods such as herbs, fruits and vegetables are gifts from mother nature. They are natural and intended to boost your immune system, help your body to heal and promote a life of longeivity.

It is very human to want to eat processed foods. However, one should try to exercise moderation-- a little of this and a little of that.

Your diet should consist of a well proportioned percentage of fruits, vegetables and herbs-- make your plate as colorful as possible.

Your skin will glow, your thought process will be clear, your hair will shine and your body will look just as good as it feels!

Always remember, prevention is better than cure and your body only performs as good as your treat it! Your body will function at its best and no one elses'!

<u>Vocabulary</u>

Ailment

Aloe

Apple

Bahamas

Bath

Blueberry

Bush

Garlic

General

Ginseng

Grape

Heal

Herb

Horseradish

Ingredient

Licorice

Lycopene

Medicine

Nomenclature

Onion

Orange

Phytochemical

<u>Useful Resources</u>

en.wikipedia.org

www.prevention.com

www.whfoods.com

www.livestrong.com

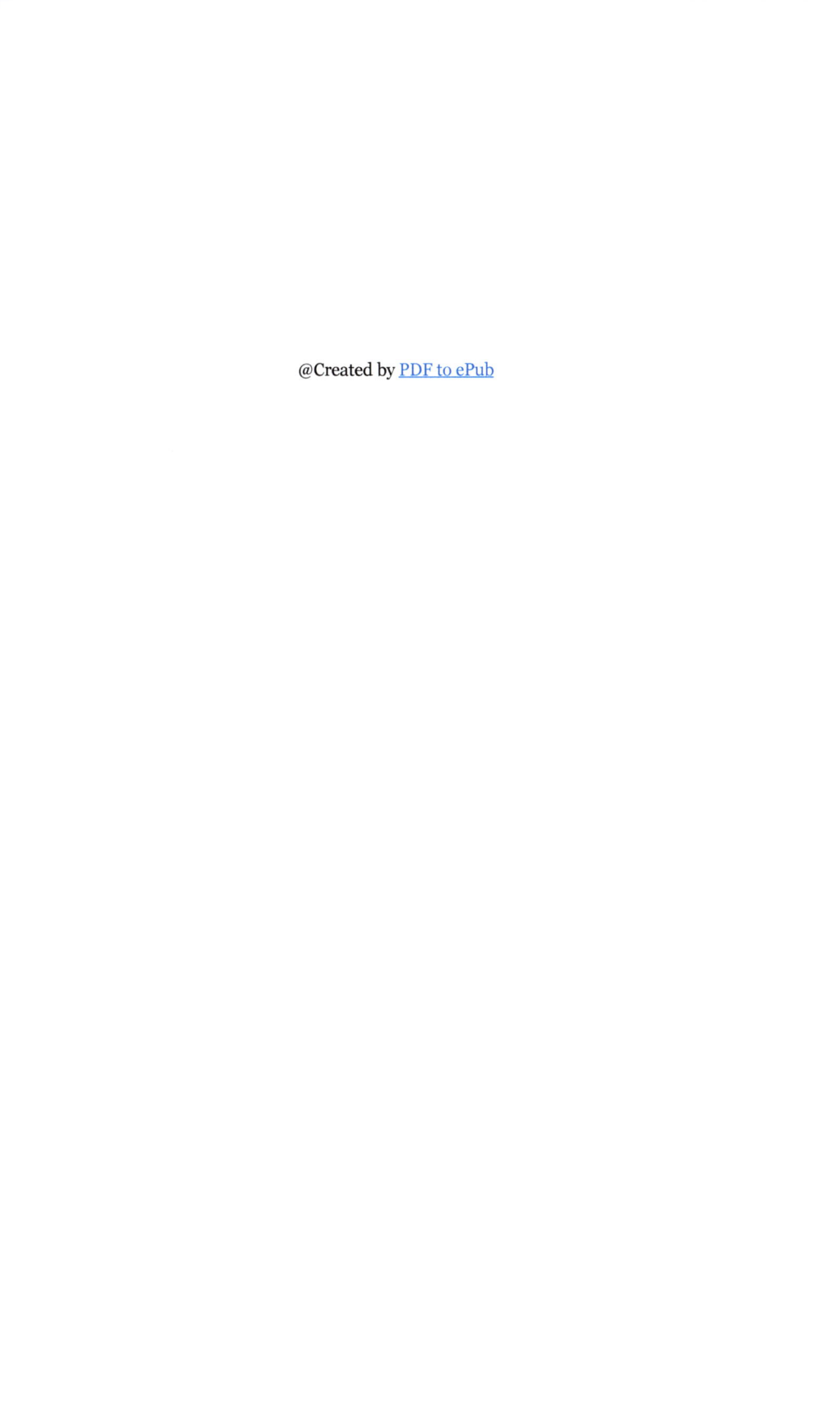
@Created by

www.ingramcontent.com/pod-product-compliance
Lightning Source LLC
Chambersburg PA
CBHW050758290526
45792CB00008B/2242